I0116179

The Rogue Librarian's Guide to Falling Asleep in 2 Minutes-- Starting Tonight!

Will Swartz

The Rogue Librarian's Guide To Falling Asleep in 2 Minutes– Starting Tonight

Copyright © 2025 by Will Swartz
All rights reserved.Published by Will Swartz Enterprises

No part of this book may be reproduced, distributed, or transmitted in any form or by any means, including photocopying, recording, or other electronic or mechanical methods, without the prior written permission of the author, except in the case of brief quotations embodied in critical reviews and certain other noncommercial uses permitted by copyright law. For permission requests, please contact the publisher at:
support@roguelibrarianpress.com

This book is a work of the author's expertise and experience. While every effort has been made to ensure the accuracy of the information presented, the author and publisher make no warranties or representations regarding its completeness or applicability. The information provided is for educational and informational purposes only and should not be considered medical, psychological, or legal advice. Readers should consult with a qualified professional for specific guidance related to their situation. The author and publisher assume no responsibility for errors, omissions, or the use or misuse of the information contained herein.

Any trademarks mentioned are the property of their respective owners and are used only for reference, without any affiliation or endorsement implied. For more information, visit Roguelibrarianpress.com

Bonus Sleep Toolkit

Hey Sleepless Reader…

Before you dive headfirst into this Rogue Rapid Read and finally get the rest you deserve (and honestly, need), I've got a gift for you.

It's called The Rogue Librarian's Sleep Toolkit, and it's completely free.
Think of it like the Swiss Army Knife of bedtime. You'll get:

- Downloadable checklists (because remembering things at bedtime is a joke)
- Worksheets to help you build your perfect sleep routine
- Tracking tools (not creepy ones, just the helpful kind)

- Links to gadgets, gear, and resources I personally recommend
- And a few delightful surprises I couldn't squeeze into this book

All of it lives on one simple, beautiful, insomnia-busting page.

Just scan this QR code to grab it

Why am I giving this away?

Because two things are true:
1. I want you to sleep better. Really. That's the whole point.

2. I'd love to send you even more Rogue wisdom, stories, and practical tools to help with sleep and other things we humans tend to mess up. No spam. Just me (and my over caffeinated brain) occasionally dropping something helpful, funny, or potentially life-improving into your inbox

So go ahead—scan the code. Get the goods.

And let's get you sleeping like a Hemingway cat.

To Noah, Noelle, Jeremy, Josiah, and Jennifer—

For every sleepless night you so generously provided, whether through midnight feedings, irrational toddler demands, or the sudden and urgent need to explain the mysteries of the universe at 2 AM. For the early morning practices that turned me into a sleep-deprived chauffeur. For the late-night games, last-minute school projects, and inexplicable bursts of energy when I was running on fumes.

You all made sure I had a front-row seat to the many ways a person can be deprived of sleep, and I'd like to think that hands-on experience gave me the credentials to write this book.

I wouldn't trade a single exhausted moment for the world (though I might have traded a few for a solid nap). You are, and always will be, my greatest adventure—even if you did rob me of a few thousand hours of rest along the way.

With love, yawns, and the eternal hope that you're all getting better sleep than I did.

—Dad

Sleep is Like a Cat

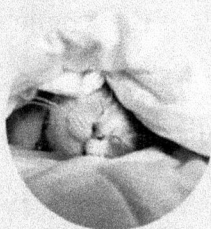

"Sleep is like a cat: It only comes to you if you ignore it." -— Gillian Flynn, Gone Girl

Table of Contents

Bonus Sleep Toolkit 4

Sleep is Like a Cat 9

From the Desk of the Rogue Librarian 13

Why Most Sleep Advice Doesn't Work
(and What Will).....................................17

How the Military Method Actually
Works 22

Try This Tonight: Your Two-Minute
Sleep Challenge....................................32

Common Mistakes and How to Avoid
Them (Without Ruining the Whole
Thing)...37

Building Your Two-Minute Sleep Habit
(Making It Stick Without Needing a
Sleep Coach in Your Closet) 44

Your Next Step: What to Do If You're
Ready for More Sleep (and More Rogue

Wisdom) 51

Notes and Sources 57

References 62

About the author 65

Nite Nite Kitty! 70

From the Desk of the Rogue Librarian

How to Fall Asleep in Two Minutes— Starting Tonight!

Let's cut to the chase.

You're tired. Not poetic, windswept, candlelit-tavern tired. No. You're real-life, eyes-gritty, thoughts-won't-stop, "why is my ceiling fan louder at 2 a.m.?" tired. The kind of tiredness that makes you question your life choices and wonder if you accidentally offended the gods of sleep somewhere around 2007.

Welcome. You're in the right place.

This is not a book of fluffy platitudes, complex jargon, or twenty-seven-point

13

plans that require Himalayan salt caves and four hours of free time you don't have.

This is a guide for people who want to fall asleep *now*. Or at least tonight. Preferably before your brain starts reminding you of that thing you said in 10th grade.

Inside these pages, you'll find something refreshingly simple: a technique that works. It's not new. It wasn't dreamed up by influencers in matching pajamas or wellness coaches with bedtime ring lights.

It came from the military—designed to help exhausted soldiers fall asleep fast, even in places where people are shooting at them. If they can do it in a war zone, you can do it in your guest bedroom surrounded by laundry and regrets. You're going to learn how to train your body to shut down on cue. Not with pills. Not with willpower. But with a method so straightforward, you'll wonder why no one taught you this before.

I'll also show you why all the other things you've tried haven't worked. Not because you're broken, or weak, or doomed to spend your nights watching the glowing numbers on the clock tick toward morning—but because most advice about sleep misses the point.

This book is short, on purpose. I don't want you reading for hours. I want you to sleep. Tonight. You can dig into my longer, more complete book later if you want the full rogue tour through insomnia's dirty tricks and the science of good sleep.

But for now, all you need is this small but mighty volume. Think of it as the librarian's contraband—smuggled out of the larger collection just for you.

So, if you're tired of being tired, if you've had enough of the bedtime struggle and the "just relax" nonsense... lean in.

I'm about to teach you how to fall asleep like a soldier—with precision, calm, and a little Rogue Librarian magic. Let's begin.

Why Most Sleep Advice Doesn't Work (and What Will)

You've probably heard this before: "Just relax. Don't think so much. Go to bed earlier."

And how's that working out?

If you're like most people with sleep problems, it's not. Because advice like that sounds helpful—until you're lying in bed at 2 a.m., staring at the ceiling, thinking about that weird noise the fridge is making or why you never learned how to fold a fitted sheet.

You don't need vague advice. You need something that actually works.

Here's the truth: sleep isn't just about being tired. It's not about trying harder. You can't force it. But you *can* train your body to fall asleep.

That's what this little book is about. It's short, because you're tired. And you need help tonight—not after five more chapters of science talk and bedtime theory.

Now, most people do the same thing when they can't sleep. They toss. They turn. They fluff the pillow, change positions, maybe scroll their phone or get up and wander the house like a well-dressed ghost.

Some people try pills. Others try tea. Or they watch a video of someone whispering into a microphone and brushing their hair for forty minutes. (Not judging. Just observing.)

But here's the problem: none of that teaches your body how to fall asleep on its own.

And the more you try, the harder it gets. You feel frustrated, maybe even broken. You wonder why this is so easy for everyone else.

But it's not. You're not the only one. You're just the only one reading this book in the dark right now.

Here's where everything changes.

During World War II, the U.S. military had a big problem. Soldiers weren't getting enough sleep. They were out in the field, under stress, trying to rest on cold ground or in loud places. And they couldn't do it. The lack of sleep was making mistakes more likely—big mistakes.

So the military came up with a solution. They created a method to teach soldiers how to fall asleep fast—under any condition. Loud or quiet. Cold or hot. Safe or stressful. It didn't matter. The goal was simple: help the body shut down and rest. On command.

It worked. And it still works today.

This method isn't hard. It takes about two minutes to learn and a little practice to master. No special tools. No perfect bedroom setup. Just a way to teach your body how to relax, step by step, until sleep comes naturally.

In the next chapter, I'll show you exactly how it works. Not with long explanations. Just a simple routine you can use tonight.

So take a deep breath. You're not broken. You're just about to learn something no one ever taught you before.

Let's go.

How the Military Method Actually Works

Alright. You've heard the hype.

A technique that supposedly knocks you out cold in two minutes flat—even in loud, uncomfortable, high-stress conditions?

Yeah, it *sounds* like one of those internet gems wedged between "this one weird trick will melt your belly fat" and "you've been brushing your teeth wrong your whole life." Except this one? Turns out—it's not total nonsense.

The method is commonly called the *Military Sleep Method*, and while its name suggests camouflage uniforms and foxholes, the truth is a little more nuanced.

Let's get that out of the way first: Despite being widely attributed to the U.S. military—specifically the Navy Pre-Flight School during World War II—there's no official military documentation confirming it was part of standardized training.

The original source? An Olympic sprint coach named Lloyd "Bud" Winter, who shared the method in his 1981 book *Relax and Win: Championship Performance*.

According to Winter, this technique was taught to help pilots fall asleep quickly under pressure, with reports claiming that 96% of them could doze off within two minutes after just six weeks of practice—even with simulated gunfire in the background.

Now, before you roll your eyes, here's the thing: While we can't verify the military's official use, the technique itself is based on legitimate relaxation strategies.

According to sources like ChoosingTherapy.com, The Sleep Doctor, Cleveland Clinic, and Verywell Mind, the method combines muscle relaxation, controlled breathing, and mental visualization—three science-backed ways to help your body and brain shift into sleep mode.

So no, it's not magic. And it doesn't involve chanting, crystals, or sleeping upside-down like a bat.

But it *is* effective—especially if you practice it consistently. It's designed to override the stress and tension that keep your brain buzzing and your body clenched like a fist.

And it's not just for soldiers or fighter pilots. If you're a civilian who's ever tried to fall asleep in a cheap hotel, a noisy apartment, or—God forbid—a red-eye flight, you're in the right place.

So here's how to begin:

First: Get comfortable. This can be your bed, your couch, a sleeping pad, the floor—whatever you've got. Soldiers practiced this sitting upright on hard chairs. You've already got an advantage. Use it.

Step 1: Relax Your Face

Start with your forehead. Soften it. That little furrow you've had since Tuesday? Let it go. Unclench your jaw. Drop your tongue from the roof of your mouth like it's just been fired. Close your eyes gently—not like you're trying to hold back a sneeze.

This alone might feel weird if you're not used to relaxing on purpose. That's okay. Keep going.

Step 2: Drop Your Shoulders

They've been pretending to be earrings all day. Let them fall. Melt them into whatever surface you're on. Imagine you're made of warm bread dough. Let it ooze. (Weird visual, but it works.)

Step 3: Let Your Arms Go Limp
Start with your hands. Let them flop like overcooked noodles. Then your forearms. Then your biceps. The goal is to feel like a puppet whose strings have all been cut. Still, calm, useless in the best possible way.

Step 4: Breathe and Sink
Take a long, slow breath. Then let it out with an exaggerated sigh, like you've just seen the price of printer ink. Feel your chest soften. Your breathing should slow down naturally. If it doesn't, just fake it until it does.

Step 5: Relax Your Legs
Same as the arms. Start at the top and work your way down. Thighs, knees, calves, ankles, feet. Everything goes soft and heavy. Like sandbags. Or, if you

prefer, like a burrito that gave up
halfway through being rolled.

Now, if you've done all that, your body
should feel heavy. Quiet. Still. Kind of
like when your dog falls asleep on the
rug and becomes immovable until there's
food involved.

Step 6: Calm the Brain

Here's the trickiest part. Your body's relaxed, but your brain? It's got opinions. So we're going to give it a job. Not a hard job. Just something boring enough to keep it busy while you drift off.

Try picturing yourself lying on a calm lake in a canoe. Sky above. Water below. No movement, no stress, no unpaid bills floating nearby. Or repeat a phrase like "I'm going to sleep now" in your mind, slowly and steadily.

If your brain tries to chime in with "What about that email you forgot to send?" just thank it politely and return to your canoe.

That's the method. Body calm. Mind quiet. Sleep incoming.

Now here's the truth: it may not work the first time. Or the second. This is a skill, not a button. Soldiers took six weeks to master it. You might get results faster— but even if you don't, keep going. Your body is listening. It just needs to learn that this routine means, "We're done for the day."

The more you use it, the faster it kicks in. It becomes muscle memory. Like tying your shoes, but in reverse. You're untying the tension in your body and signaling to your brain: time to power down.

And remember—this works even if your room isn't silent, your sheets aren't perfect, or your spouse is snoring like a chainsaw. It's not about perfect conditions. It's about *training the system*.

Try it tonight. Stick with it. You'll be surprised how quickly your body responds.

Next up? Your two-minute challenge.

Let's turn this method into a routine—and see what happens when you actually give your body permission to sleep.

Turn the page. We're just getting started.

Try This Tonight: Your Two-Minute Sleep Challenge

Alright, you've made it this far.

You've read about the Military Method. You've nodded along. Maybe you even flopped your arms around a bit in your chair to see if you could feel like overcooked spaghetti. That's good. That means you're ready.

Now it's time to actually do it.

Tonight, I'm inviting you to a challenge. A small one. No medals. No boot camp yelling. No pushups. Just you, your pillow, and a body that's ready to learn something new.

Here's how it works:

When you're ready for bed, set yourself up like usual—brush your teeth, turn off the lights, do whatever end-of-day rituals make you feel slightly more human. Then, when you're in bed, take a moment. Don't scroll. Don't check one last thing. Don't try to "earn" sleep by worrying about tomorrow's to-do list.

Just pause. Then walk through the Military Method. One step at a time. Don't rush it.

Start with your face. Let it soften.

Then your shoulders, arms, chest, legs. Let everything melt into the mattress. Take that big sigh. Let it all go.

When your body feels still and heavy—
like you've been turned into a sleep
burrito—it's time to give your brain
something gentle to do.

**Picture that peaceful scene, repeat that
sleepy phrase, or breathe slowly while
counting backwards from 10.**

If a thought shows up (and one probably
will), don't fight it. Just nod at it like a
neighbor walking by your house and
return to your calm scene.

Now, here's the secret sauce: if it doesn't
work instantly, don't panic. Don't tense
up. Don't declare the method a failure
and reach for your phone. Just reset. Go
back to your breath. Start again if you
want to. That's part of the training.

Because this isn't about falling asleep *once*. It's about retraining your whole system—body and mind—to know what to do when you say, "It's bedtime."
And that takes practice. Soldiers who mastered this method didn't do it in one night. They did it night after night, teaching their bodies that this routine meant one thing: lights out.

So tonight, your challenge is simple: try it. No pressure. No expectations. Just practice.

Do it again tomorrow. And again the next night. Track what happens. See how long it takes. Watch for the moment it clicks.

Because once it does, you'll realize something amazing. You don't have to *fight* sleep anymore.

You can *invite* it.

And sleep, when it finally trusts you again, will show up.

So take the challenge tonight. Turn off the lights. Relax your face. Sink into the mattress like you belong there (because you do). And let your brain know: the war is over. We're safe now. We can rest.

Two minutes. That's all it takes.

Let's get to work.

Common Mistakes and How to Avoid Them (Without Ruining the Whole Thing)

So you tried the Military Method.

You closed your eyes, relaxed your face, turned your arms into wet noodles, and floated yourself off to that quiet lake in your mind.

And then... you stared at the ceiling. Again.

If that happens, don't worry. It doesn't mean you broke it. You didn't fail the test. There is no test. Sleep isn't graded on a curve, and you don't get kicked out of the club for not drifting off like a soldier in a hammock on night one.

It just means you might've hit one of the common landmines.

Let's talk about those.

Mistake #1: Expecting It to Work Instantly

Yes, the method is fast. Yes, it was designed to help people fall asleep in two minutes. But here's the fine print nobody reads: *that's after practice*. Soldiers trained with this method every night for six weeks.

This isn't a magic switch—it's more like muscle memory. You're teaching your body, "Hey, when we do these steps, it's time to shut down."

And like anything you train, it takes reps. It's okay if you're still a little twitchy on night three. That's normal. Keep going.

Mistake #2: Rushing Through the Steps

This one's sneaky. You start off well, then halfway through relaxing your arms, you think, *"Okay, I'm relaxed, now sleep already!"* That's not how it works.

If you're rushing through it like a kid trying to finish their chores before cartoons, your body knows. You have to actually let go. Really let go. Sink. Melt. Drift. This is not the time for multitasking or mental checklists.

Be patient. Go slow. Trust the process. Your nervous system needs time to shift gears.

Mistake #3: Using It in a Bad Sleep Environment

I know we said this method works "anywhere." And it does. But that doesn't mean you should be trying it while blasting YouTube videos in a room lit up like a dentist's office, under a weighted blanket that feels like a collapsing tent. Help yourself out.

Turn off the bright lights. Lower the noise. Make the room cooler (your body sleeps better that way). You don't need perfection, but you do need peace.

If your sleep space is working *against* you, even a great method like this will be pushing uphill.

Mistake #4: Letting Your Brain Hijack the Whole Thing

You relax your body. Everything feels heavy and quiet. And then your brain shows up like, *"Hey, remember that weird thing you said to your boss four years ago?"*

Yep. Classic.

The mistake isn't that thoughts come. That's normal. The mistake is following them. Grabbing hold. Letting one worry lead to another like a conga line of mental chaos.

You don't need to *fight* your thoughts— you just don't invite them in for tea.

When a thought shows up, nod at it like a passing squirrel and go back to your calm place. Re-anchor. Breathe. Reset.

That's part of the method too

Mistake #5: Giving Up Too Soon
Let me say it again: this is a skill. You wouldn't give up on learning guitar because you didn't shred a solo on day two. So don't give up on sleep because night one didn't turn you into a bedtime ninja.

Stick with it. Night after night. You're building something powerful— something your body will come to trust.

Because when it works—and it *will*— you won't just fall asleep faster. You'll *know* how to fall asleep. On purpose. On command. Even when life is noisy, stressful, or just plain uncooperative.

And that, my friend, is the kind of superpower worth building.

Now that you know what to avoid, it's time to keep moving forward. In the next chapter, I'm going to give you a few practical tools to help you turn this method into a real habit—not just a thing you tried once after brushing your teeth. Ready for your next move?

Let's go.

Building Your Two-Minute Sleep Habit (Making It Stick Without Needing a Sleep Coach in Your Closet)

Here's the thing about sleep tricks: they're fun when they work. They feel like a little win. Like finding five bucks in your jeans pocket or realizing your leftovers didn't go bad.

But what are you building here? This isn't a trick.

This is a habit.

A repeatable, reliable, "my body knows what to do" routine that tells your nervous system, every single night: *It's okay to let go now. We're done.*

And if you want this method to actually change your life—and not just be a random thing you tried once next to an open bag of tortilla chips—you've got to build it into your routine.

Don't panic. I'm not talking about a 12-step bedtime boot camp with color-coded charts and a singing bowl.

I'm talking about one small, powerful move: do it *every night*.

It doesn't need to be perfect. It doesn't need to be fancy. You just need to do it again.

Why? Because your brain and body love patterns. They're wired for rhythm and routine. It's how you know which drawer the forks are in and which sock goes on which foot. Repetition teaches your brain, *"This comes next."*

So the more you do this method, the more your system starts linking it to sleep. You won't even have to try so hard. You'll relax your face and your body will say, "Ah, I know what this is. Time to shut down."

Pretty soon, it becomes automatic.

And then? You've got yourself a sleep switch. Not a trick. A skill. A habit.

"But What If I Miss a Night?"
Then you miss a night.

You don't throw away your toothbrush because you forgot to brush once. You don't give up walking because you tripped over the dog. Missing a night is just that—*missing a night*.

No guilt. No spiral. Just come back to it the next night like a grown-up with a plan.

The Power of a Cue

Here's a little habit-building bonus: link this method to something you *already do* before bed.

Maybe it's brushing your teeth. Maybe it's putting your phone down (or tossing it across the room if you're dramatic like me). Maybe it's turning off the last light in the house and mumbling "we survived another day."

Whatever it is, let that action be your cue. That's the moment you shift from the day's chaos to the sleep routine.

The cue tells your brain, "Okay, the show's over. Curtains down."

Make It Yours
Some people like using a calm mental picture. Others repeat a sleepy phrase in their head. Some might pray, meditate, or just breathe slowly while pretending their bed is a canoe.

You do *not* have to do it my way. You're not trying to become the Rogue Librarian. (One of me is enough, ask my family.)

You're trying to become the well-rested version of *you*. So tweak the practice. Shape it. Give it your own flavor. The steps work—but the style is yours to choose.

Because what you're building is more than just better sleep.

You're building control. You're saying, "Hey brain, I've got this now."
You're learning how to tell your body when to let go. When to stop bracing. When to fall into rest without a fight.

And, when that habit sticks, you'll never look at sleep the same way again. You'll *own* it.

Now, before we wrap this up, let's talk about what's next.

Because for some of you, this pocket guide might be all you need. But for others? You might be curious about what else is possible—and how deep this rabbit hole of better sleep goes.

Let's take a quick peek at that together.
Turn the page. We're almost there.

Your Next Step: What to Do If You're Ready for More Sleep (and More Rogue Wisdom)

If you've made it to this chapter, congratulations: You've read the whole book. A short one, sure. But you didn't skim it, you didn't quit halfway through, and you didn't fall asleep on page two (though, in this particular case, that would've actually been a win).

More importantly—you showed up. You gave sleep another chance. You tried something new. You didn't just accept that you were "bad at sleeping" or "just wired this way." You pushed back.

And that makes you the kind of person I like.

You're probably already noticing a shift. Maybe you've had your first two-minute success. Or maybe you're just starting to feel more calm, more in control, more like *you're* the one driving this sleep bus —not your stress, not your screen, and definitely not that voice in your head that gets chatty at midnight.

Now, here's the honest part:This method works. But it's not the whole story.

Falling asleep quickly is one piece of the puzzle. But what about staying asleep? What about the nights when your body feels tired but your brain turns into a late-night talk show host? What about the things you're doing during the day that are messing with your nights without you even realizing it?

That's why I wrote the *full* book:

The Rogue Librarian's Guide to Sleep —Real Help for Insomnia

It's everything I've learned after years of research, experiments, failures, sleep studies, CPAP battles, late-night snacks I regretted, and figuring out what actually works.

It covers:
- How to fix your sleep environment (without needing a designer headboard)
- What to eat (and *when*) to help—not hurt—your sleep
- How movement during the day rewires your night
- What to do when your brain won't stop spinning

- Why modern life wrecks your sleep—and how to take it back
- How to fall asleep, stay asleep, and wake up feeling like a halfway functional human being again

All of it in my voice, with a little humor, a lot of help, and zero fluff.
If this short guide helped you, then the full book is your next step.More tools. More strategies. More rogue wisdom. More peace. More sleep.

You can buy it on Amazon or direct from me by scanning the QR code below:

And if you want the bonus tools—sleep trackers, routines, checklists, scent experiments, and more—I've bundled them all into one handy place:

All free. No strings. No spam. Just good stuff to help you sleep like you were *meant to.* Because friend, sleep is not a luxury. It's not a reward. It's a basic human need—and it's time you got yours back.

So keep going. You're not stuck. You're not broken. You're just getting started. Now turn off the light. You've got this.

Endless summer,

Will
The Rogue Librarian

https://linktr.ee/wswartz

Notes and Sources

Origins and Military Use

The method is widely attributed to Lloyd "Bud" Winter, an Olympic sprint coach who documented it in his 1981 book *Relax and Win: Championship Performance*. Winter claimed that the U.S. Navy Pre-Flight School developed this technique during World War II to help pilots fall asleep quickly under stressful conditions. According to the book, after six weeks of practice, 96% of pilots could reportedly fall asleep within two minutes, even amidst distractions like gunfire.

However, there is no publicly available military documentation or peer-reviewed research confirming that this method was officially taught or used by the military.

While it's plausible that such techniques were informally shared among service members, definitive evidence is lacking.

Technique Overview

The Military Sleep Method involves a series of steps aimed at promoting relaxation:

- **Relax the Face**: Close your eyes and consciously relax all facial muscles, including the jaw, tongue, and muscles around the eyes.
- **Drop the Shoulders and Arms**: Let your shoulders drop as low as possible, followed by relaxing each arm, one at a time.
- **Exhale and Relax the Chest**: Breathe out slowly, allowing your chest to relax.

- **Relax the Legs**: Starting from the thighs, consciously relax each part of your legs down to your feet.
- **Clear the Mind**: Spend about 10 seconds clearing your mind. Visualization techniques, such as imagining lying in a canoe on a calm lake, can be helpful. If intrusive thoughts persist, repeating the phrase "don't think" for 10 seconds may assist in achieving mental calmness

Scientific Evaluation

While the Military Sleep Method itself hasn't been subjected to rigorous scientific studies, the techniques it employs are grounded in well-researched relaxation practices:

- **Progressive Muscle Relaxation (PMR)**: This involves systematically tensing and then

relaxing different muscle groups,
which has been shown to reduce
anxiety and improve sleep quality
.

- **Deep Breathing**: Slow, deep
  breathing activates the
  parasympathetic nervous system,
  promoting a state of calm
  conducive to sleep.
- **Visualization**: Imagining
  peaceful scenes can distract from
  stressful thoughts and facilitate
  relaxation.

Experts, including Dr. Alaina Tiani from
the Cleveland Clinic, acknowledge that
while these components are beneficial,
the claim of falling asleep within two
minutes may not be realistic for
everyone. The effectiveness of such
techniques can vary based on individual
differences and consistency of practice.

Conclusion

The Military Sleep Method integrates established relaxation techniques that can aid in falling asleep more quickly. Although its purported military origins lack concrete evidence, the method's components are supported by scientific research on sleep and relaxation. While it may not guarantee sleep within two minutes for everyone, consistent practice of these techniques can contribute to improved sleep quality over time.

References

Works Cited
Note: URLs are provided for reference. Readers may need to enter them manually to access the original sources.

Big Think. "The 5-Step 'Military Method' for Falling Asleep in Minutes." *Big Think*, 2023. www.bigthink.com/health/military-method-sleep/. Accessed 15 May 2025.

Cleveland Clinic. "The Military Sleep Method: Does It Work?" *Cleveland Clinic Health Essentials*, 2023. Accessed 15 May 2025.

Good Housekeeping. "Can't Fall Asleep? The Military Sleep Method Claims to Help You Drift Off in Minutes." *Good Housekeeping*, 2023. Accessed 15 May 2025.

Healthline. "How to Fall Asleep Fast in 10, 60, or 120 Seconds." *Healthline*, 2023. Accessed 15 May 2025.

Sleep Doctor. "Military Sleep Method: How It Works." *Sleep Doctor*, 2023. www.sleepdoctor.com/sleep-hygiene/ military-sleep-method/. Accessed 15 May 2025.

Sleepopolis. "I Tried the Military Sleep Method: Here's How It Went." *Sleepopolis*, 2023. www.sleepopolis.com/blog/military-sleep-method/. Accessed 15 May 2025.

University of Minnesota Medical School. "Practice the Military Sleep Method to Fall Asleep in Mere Minutes." *University of Minnesota Medical School News*, 2023. med.umn.edu/news-events/ military-sleep-method. Accessed 15 May 2025.

Verywell Mind. "The Military Sleep
Method: Benefits and How It Works."
Verywell Mind, 2023.
www.verywellmind.com/military-sleep-
method-7480441. Accessed 15 May
2025.

About the author

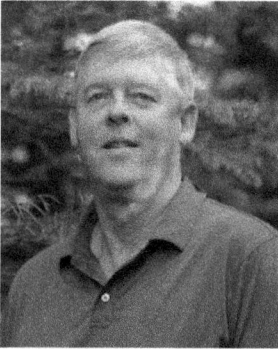

After 35 years as a teacher, librarian, administrator, coach, and professional wearer of many hats (some more stylish than others), I did what every weary educator dreams of during standardized testing week: I retired.

But let's be clear—retirement for me wasn't a surrender to rocking chairs and reruns. It was more of a personal commencement ceremony. While my students tossed caps in the air, I tossed my briefcase in the closet and asked myself, "Whatta ya wanna do today?"

My answer: everything.

Armed with six decades of stories, scars, and a slightly overstuffed backpack, I headed to the woods—not in the sit-and-muse-like-Thoreau sense, but the hike-from-Lake-Huron-to-Lake-Michigan kind of way. I wanted to live deliberately, seek the essential, and wring every drop of meaning from this next chapter.

Before all that, I served students across Michigan and China as an English and Spanish teacher, librarian, basketball coach, alternative ed principal, tech trainer, preschool director, and district administrator.

I've taught in classrooms, coached on courts, and even co-wrangled an 800-kid preschool program (no small feat, trust me).

My formal credentials include a B.A. in English/Spanish, a Master's in Library and Information Science, and a certificate in Educational Technology—but most of my real education has come from the trail, the classroom, and the occasional parenting misadventure.

Today, I'm a writer, traveler, speaker, and perpetual learner. I write books, build online resources, hike long trails, and help people wrestle meaning out of life's chaos.

Whether I'm creating tools to help hikers prepare for the backcountry, guides to help readers sleep better, or humorous tales from my years in education, my goal is the same: leave the world a little more inspired—and maybe a little better rested—than I found it.

I believe the best chapters are still ahead. Let's walk there together.

Nite Nite Kitty!

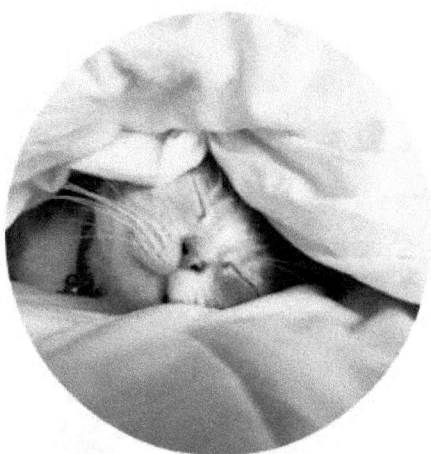

www.ingramcontent.com/pod-product-compliance
Lightning Source LLC
Chambersburg PA
CBHW060519280326
41933CB00014B/3036